Copyright 2016, Mega Media Depot
Published by Mega Media Depot
Manufactured in the United States of America
All rights reserved.

P.O. Box 945
Prospect Heights, Il 60070

Introduction

Thank you for purchasing our daily diet log!

This Diet Journal is a deluxe food diary with plenty of room to record quantities and food counts (calories, fat, carbs, protein, etc.) of breakfast, lunch, dinner, and snacks. A special area for daily totals makes it easy to see at a glance how you are doing.

What makes this Diet Journal special is that we have included 108 pages to keep you on track. This is a great way to stay motivated!

This Diet Journal can be used with virtually any food or fitness program. It has been proven that keeping a food journal helps people focus and stay more committed to improving their eating habits. It really works!

FOOD	QTY	CALS	CARBS	PRO (g)	FAT (g)

BREAKFAST

	Sub Total				

LUNCH

	Sub Total				

DINNER

	Sub Total				

SNACK

	Sub Total				
	Total				

NUTRIENT	TOTAL	UNITS	GOAL %	RDA%
Calories				
Fat				
Saturated Fat				
Polyunsaturated				
Monounsaturated				

FOOD	QTY	CALS	CARBS	PRO (g)	FAT (g)

BREAKFAST

	Sub Total				

LUNCH

	Sub Total				

DINNER

	Sub Total				

SNACK

	Sub Total				
	Total				

NUTRIENT	TOTAL	UNITS	GOAL %	RDA%
Calories				
Fat				
Saturated Fat				
Polyunsaturated				
Monounsaturated				

FOOD	QTY	CALS	CARBS	PRO (g)	FAT (g)

BREAKFAST

	Sub Total				

LUNCH

	Sub Total				

DINNER

	Sub Total				

SNACK

	Sub Total				
	Total				

NUTRIENT	TOTAL	UNITS	GOAL %	RDA%
Calories				
Fat				
Saturated Fat				
Polyunsaturated				
Monounsaturated				

FOOD	QTY	CALS	CARBS	PRO (g)	FAT (g)

BREAKFAST

		Sub Total			

LUNCH

		Sub Total			

DINNER

		Sub Total			

SNACK

		Sub Total			
		Total			

NUTRIENT	TOTAL	UNITS	GOAL %	RDA%
Calories				
Fat				
Saturated Fat				
Polyunsaturated				
Monounsaturated				

FOOD	QTY	CALS	CARBS	PRO (g)	FAT (g)

BREAKFAST

	Sub Total				

LUNCH

	Sub Total				

DINNER

	Sub Total				

SNACK

	Sub Total				
	Total				

NUTRIENT	TOTAL	UNITS	GOAL %	RDA%
Calories				
Fat				
Saturated Fat				
Polyunsaturated				
Monounsaturated				

FOOD	QTY	CALS	CARBS	PRO (g)	FAT (g)

BREAKFAST

	Sub Total				

LUNCH

	Sub Total				

DINNER

	Sub Total				

SNACK

	Sub Total				
	Total				

NUTRIENT	TOTAL	UNITS	GOAL %	RDA%
Calories				
Fat				
Saturated Fat				
Polyunsaturated				
Monounsaturated				

FOOD	QTY	CALS	CARBS	PRO (g)	FAT (g)

BREAKFAST

FOOD	QTY	CALS	CARBS	PRO (g)	FAT (g)
	Sub Total				

LUNCH

FOOD	QTY	CALS	CARBS	PRO (g)	FAT (g)
	Sub Total				

DINNER

FOOD	QTY	CALS	CARBS	PRO (g)	FAT (g)
	Sub Total				

SNACK

FOOD	QTY	CALS	CARBS	PRO (g)	FAT (g)
	Sub Total				
	Total				

NUTRIENT	TOTAL	UNITS	GOAL %	RDA%
Calories				
Fat				
Saturated Fat				
Polyunsaturated				
Monounsaturated				

FOOD	QTY	CALS	CARBS	PRO (g)	FAT (g)

BREAKFAST

	Sub Total				

LUNCH

	Sub Total				

DINNER

	Sub Total				

SNACK

	Sub Total				
	Total				

NUTRIENT	TOTAL	UNITS	GOAL %	RDA%
Calories				
Fat				
Saturated Fat				
Polyunsaturated				
Monounsaturated				

FOOD	QTY	CALS	CARBS	PRO (g)	FAT (g)

BREAKFAST

	Sub Total				

LUNCH

	Sub Total				

DINNER

	Sub Total				

SNACK

	Sub Total				
	Total				

NUTRIENT	TOTAL	UNITS	GOAL %	RDA%
Calories				
Fat				
Saturated Fat				
Polyunsaturated				
Monounsaturated				

FOOD	QTY	CALS	CARBS	PRO (g)	FAT (g)

BREAKFAST

FOOD	QTY	CALS	CARBS	PRO (g)	FAT (g)
	Sub Total				

LUNCH

FOOD	QTY	CALS	CARBS	PRO (g)	FAT (g)
	Sub Total				

DINNER

FOOD	QTY	CALS	CARBS	PRO (g)	FAT (g)
	Sub Total				

SNACK

FOOD	QTY	CALS	CARBS	PRO (g)	FAT (g)
	Sub Total				
	Total				

NUTRIENT	TOTAL	UNITS	GOAL %	RDA%
Calories				
Fat				
Saturated Fat				
Polyunsaturated				
Monounsaturated				

FOOD	QTY	CALS	CARBS	PRO (g)	FAT (g)

BREAKFAST

	Sub Total				

LUNCH

	Sub Total				

DINNER

	Sub Total				

SNACK

	Sub Total				
	Total				

NUTRIENT	TOTAL	UNITS	GOAL %	RDA%
Calories				
Fat				
Saturated Fat				
Polyunsaturated				
Monounsaturated				

FOOD	QTY	CALS	CARBS	PRO (g)	FAT (g)

BREAKFAST

	Sub Total				

LUNCH

	Sub Total				

DINNER

	Sub Total				

SNACK

	Sub Total				
	Total				

NUTRIENT	TOTAL	UNITS	GOAL %	RDA%
Calories				
Fat				
Saturated Fat				
Polyunsaturated				
Monounsaturated				

FOOD	QTY	CALS	CARBS	PRO (g)	FAT (g)

BREAKFAST

	Sub Total				

LUNCH

	Sub Total				

DINNER

	Sub Total				

SNACK

	Sub Total				
	Total				

NUTRIENT	TOTAL	UNITS	GOAL %	RDA%
Calories				
Fat				
Saturated Fat				
Polyunsaturated				
Monounsaturated				

FOOD	QTY	CALS	CARBS	PRO (g)	FAT (g)

BREAKFAST

	Sub Total				

LUNCH

	Sub Total				

DINNER

	Sub Total				

SNACK

	Sub Total				
	Total				

NUTRIENT	TOTAL	UNITS	GOAL %	RDA%
Calories				
Fat				
Saturated Fat				
Polyunsaturated				
Monounsaturated				

FOOD	QTY	CALS	CARBS	PRO (g)	FAT (g)

BREAKFAST

	Sub Total				

LUNCH

	Sub Total				

DINNER

	Sub Total				

SNACK

	Sub Total				
	Total				

NUTRIENT	TOTAL	UNITS	GOAL %	RDA%
Calories				
Fat				
Saturated Fat				
Polyunsaturated				
Monounsaturated				

FOOD	QTY	CALS	CARBS	PRO (g)	FAT (g)

BREAKFAST

	Sub Total				

LUNCH

	Sub Total				

DINNER

	Sub Total				

SNACK

	Sub Total				
	Total				

NUTRIENT	TOTAL	UNITS	GOAL %	RDA%
Calories				
Fat				
Saturated Fat				
Polyunsaturated				
Monounsaturated				

FOOD	QTY	CALS	CARBS	PRO (g)	FAT (g)

BREAKFAST

	Sub Total				

LUNCH

	Sub Total				

DINNER

	Sub Total				

SNACK

	Sub Total				
	Total				

NUTRIENT	TOTAL	UNITS	GOAL %	RDA%
Calories				
Fat				
Saturated Fat				
Polyunsaturated				
Monounsaturated				

FOOD	QTY	CALS	CARBS	PRO (g)	FAT (g)

BREAKFAST

	Sub Total				

LUNCH

	Sub Total				

DINNER

	Sub Total				

SNACK

	Sub Total				
	Total				

NUTRIENT	TOTAL	UNITS	GOAL %	RDA%
Calories				
Fat				
Saturated Fat				
Polyunsaturated				
Monounsaturated				

FOOD	QTY	CALS	CARBS	PRO (g)	FAT (g)

BREAKFAST

	Sub Total				

LUNCH

	Sub Total				

DINNER

	Sub Total				

SNACK

	Sub Total				
	Total				

NUTRIENT	TOTAL	UNITS	GOAL %	RDA%
Calories				
Fat				
Saturated Fat				
Polyunsaturated				
Monounsaturated				

FOOD	QTY	CALS	CARBS	PRO (g)	FAT (g)

BREAKFAST

	Sub Total				

LUNCH

	Sub Total				

DINNER

	Sub Total				

SNACK

	Sub Total				
	Total				

NUTRIENT	TOTAL	UNITS	GOAL %	RDA%
Calories				
Fat				
Saturated Fat				
Polyunsaturated				
Monounsaturated				

FOOD	QTY	CALS	CARBS	PRO (g)	FAT (g)

BREAKFAST

	Sub Total				

LUNCH

	Sub Total				

DINNER

	Sub Total				

SNACK

	Sub Total				
	Total				

NUTRIENT	TOTAL	UNITS	GOAL %	RDA%
Calories				
Fat				
Saturated Fat				
Polyunsaturated				
Monounsaturated				

FOOD	QTY	CALS	CARBS	PRO (g)	FAT (g)

BREAKFAST

	Sub Total				

LUNCH

	Sub Total				

DINNER

	Sub Total				

SNACK

	Sub Total				
	Total				

NUTRIENT	TOTAL	UNITS	GOAL %	RDA%
Calories				
Fat				
Saturated Fat				
Polyunsaturated				
Monounsaturated				

FOOD	QTY	CALS	CARBS	PRO (g)	FAT (g)

BREAKFAST

	Sub Total				

LUNCH

	Sub Total				

DINNER

	Sub Total				

SNACK

	Sub Total				
	Total				

NUTRIENT	TOTAL	UNITS	GOAL %	RDA%
Calories				
Fat				
Saturated Fat				
Polyunsaturated				
Monounsaturated				

FOOD	QTY	CALS	CARBS	PRO (g)	FAT (g)

BREAKFAST

	Sub Total				

LUNCH

	Sub Total				

DINNER

	Sub Total				

SNACK

	Sub Total				
	Total				

NUTRIENT	TOTAL	UNITS	GOAL %	RDA%
Calories				
Fat				
Saturated Fat				
Polyunsaturated				
Monounsaturated				

FOOD	QTY	CALS	CARBS	PRO (g)	FAT (g)

BREAKFAST

	Sub Total				

LUNCH

	Sub Total				

DINNER

	Sub Total				

SNACK

	Sub Total				
	Total				

NUTRIENT	TOTAL	UNITS	GOAL %	RDA%
Calories				
Fat				
Saturated Fat				
Polyunsaturated				
Monounsaturated				

FOOD	QTY	CALS	CARBS	PRO (g)	FAT (g)

BREAKFAST

	Sub Total				

LUNCH

	Sub Total				

DINNER

	Sub Total				

SNACK

	Sub Total				
	Total				

NUTRIENT	TOTAL	UNITS	GOAL %	RDA%
Calories				
Fat				
Saturated Fat				
Polyunsaturated				
Monounsaturated				

FOOD	QTY	CALS	CARBS	PRO (g)	FAT (g)

BREAKFAST

	Sub Total				

LUNCH

	Sub Total				

DINNER

	Sub Total				

SNACK

	Sub Total				
	Total				

NUTRIENT	TOTAL	UNITS	GOAL %	RDA%
Calories				
Fat				
Saturated Fat				
Polyunsaturated				
Monounsaturated				

FOOD	QTY	CALS	CARBS	PRO (g)	FAT (g)

BREAKFAST

	Sub Total				

LUNCH

	Sub Total				

DINNER

	Sub Total				

SNACK

	Sub Total				
	Total				

NUTRIENT	TOTAL	UNITS	GOAL %	RDA%
Calories				
Fat				
Saturated Fat				
Polyunsaturated				
Monounsaturated				

FOOD	QTY	CALS	CARBS	PRO (g)	FAT (g)

BREAKFAST

	Sub Total				

LUNCH

	Sub Total				

DINNER

	Sub Total				

SNACK

	Sub Total				
	Total				

NUTRIENT	TOTAL	UNITS	GOAL %	RDA%
Calories				
Fat				
Saturated Fat				
Polyunsaturated				
Monounsaturated				

FOOD	QTY	CALS	CARBS	PRO (g)	FAT (g)

BREAKFAST

	Sub Total				

LUNCH

	Sub Total				

DINNER

	Sub Total				

SNACK

	Sub Total				
	Total				

NUTRIENT	TOTAL	UNITS	GOAL %	RDA%
Calories				
Fat				
Saturated Fat				
Polyunsaturated				
Monounsaturated				

FOOD	QTY	CALS	CARBS	PRO (g)	FAT (g)

BREAKFAST

		Sub Total			

LUNCH

		Sub Total			

DINNER

		Sub Total			

SNACK

		Sub Total			
		Total			

NUTRIENT	TOTAL	UNITS	GOAL %	RDA%
Calories				
Fat				
Saturated Fat				
Polyunsaturated				
Monounsaturated				

FOOD	QTY	CALS	CARBS	PRO (g)	FAT (g)

BREAKFAST

	Sub Total				

LUNCH

	Sub Total				

DINNER

	Sub Total				

SNACK

	Sub Total				
	Total				

NUTRIENT	TOTAL	UNITS	GOAL %	RDA%
Calories				
Fat				
Saturated Fat				
Polyunsaturated				
Monounsaturated				

FOOD	QTY	CALS	CARBS	PRO (g)	FAT (g)

BREAKFAST

	Sub Total				

LUNCH

	Sub Total				

DINNER

	Sub Total				

SNACK

	Sub Total				
	Total				

NUTRIENT	TOTAL	UNITS	GOAL %	RDA%
Calories				
Fat				
Saturated Fat				
Polyunsaturated				
Monounsaturated				

FOOD	QTY	CALS	CARBS	PRO (g)	FAT (g)

BREAKFAST

FOOD	QTY	CALS	CARBS	PRO (g)	FAT (g)
	Sub Total				

LUNCH

FOOD	QTY	CALS	CARBS	PRO (g)	FAT (g)
	Sub Total				

DINNER

FOOD	QTY	CALS	CARBS	PRO (g)	FAT (g)
	Sub Total				

SNACK

FOOD	QTY	CALS	CARBS	PRO (g)	FAT (g)
	Sub Total				
	Total				

NUTRIENT	TOTAL	UNITS	GOAL %	RDA%
Calories				
Fat				
Saturated Fat				
Polyunsaturated				
Monounsaturated				

FOOD	QTY	CALS	CARBS	PRO (g)	FAT (g)

BREAKFAST

	Sub Total				

LUNCH

	Sub Total				

DINNER

	Sub Total				

SNACK

	Sub Total				
	Total				

NUTRIENT	TOTAL	UNITS	GOAL %	RDA%
Calories				
Fat				
Saturated Fat				
Polyunsaturated				
Monounsaturated				

FOOD	QTY	CALS	CARBS	PRO (g)	FAT (g)

BREAKFAST

	Sub Total				

LUNCH

	Sub Total				

DINNER

	Sub Total				

SNACK

	Sub Total				
	Total				

NUTRIENT	TOTAL	UNITS	GOAL %	RDA%
Calories				
Fat				
Saturated Fat				
Polyunsaturated				
Monounsaturated				

FOOD	QTY	CALS	CARBS	PRO (g)	FAT (g)

BREAKFAST

FOOD	QTY	CALS	CARBS	PRO (g)	FAT (g)
	Sub Total				

LUNCH

FOOD	QTY	CALS	CARBS	PRO (g)	FAT (g)
	Sub Total				

DINNER

FOOD	QTY	CALS	CARBS	PRO (g)	FAT (g)
	Sub Total				

SNACK

FOOD	QTY	CALS	CARBS	PRO (g)	FAT (g)
	Sub Total				
	Total				

NUTRIENT	TOTAL	UNITS	GOAL %	RDA%
Calories				
Fat				
Saturated Fat				
Polyunsaturated				
Monounsaturated				

FOOD	QTY	CALS	CARBS	PRO (g)	FAT (g)

BREAKFAST

		Sub Total			

LUNCH

		Sub Total			

DINNER

		Sub Total			

SNACK

		Sub Total			
		Total			

NUTRIENT	TOTAL	UNITS	GOAL %	RDA%
Calories				
Fat				
Saturated Fat				
Polyunsaturated				
Monounsaturated				

FOOD	QTY	CALS	CARBS	PRO (g)	FAT (g)

BREAKFAST

FOOD	QTY	CALS	CARBS	PRO (g)	FAT (g)
	Sub Total				

LUNCH

FOOD	QTY	CALS	CARBS	PRO (g)	FAT (g)
	Sub Total				

DINNER

FOOD	QTY	CALS	CARBS	PRO (g)	FAT (g)
	Sub Total				

SNACK

FOOD	QTY	CALS	CARBS	PRO (g)	FAT (g)
	Sub Total				
	Total				

NUTRIENT	TOTAL	UNITS	GOAL %	RDA%
Calories				
Fat				
Saturated Fat				
Polyunsaturated				
Monounsaturated				

FOOD	QTY	CALS	CARBS	PRO (g)	FAT (g)

BREAKFAST

	Sub Total				

LUNCH

	Sub Total				

DINNER

	Sub Total				

SNACK

	Sub Total				
	Total				

NUTRIENT	TOTAL	UNITS	GOAL %	RDA%
Calories				
Fat				
Saturated Fat				
Polyunsaturated				
Monounsaturated				

FOOD	QTY	CALS	CARBS	PRO (g)	FAT (g)

BREAKFAST

	Sub Total				

LUNCH

	Sub Total				

DINNER

	Sub Total				

SNACK

	Sub Total				
	Total				

NUTRIENT	TOTAL	UNITS	GOAL %	RDA%
Calories				
Fat				
Saturated Fat				
Polyunsaturated				
Monounsaturated				

FOOD	QTY	CALS	CARBS	PRO (g)	FAT (g)

BREAKFAST

	Sub Total				

LUNCH

	Sub Total				

DINNER

	Sub Total				

SNACK

	Sub Total				
	Total				

NUTRIENT	TOTAL	UNITS	GOAL %	RDA%
Calories				
Fat				
Saturated Fat				
Polyunsaturated				
Monounsaturated				

FOOD	QTY	CALS	CARBS	PRO (g)	FAT (g)

BREAKFAST

FOOD	QTY	CALS	CARBS	PRO (g)	FAT (g)
	Sub Total				

LUNCH

FOOD	QTY	CALS	CARBS	PRO (g)	FAT (g)
	Sub Total				

DINNER

FOOD	QTY	CALS	CARBS	PRO (g)	FAT (g)
	Sub Total				

SNACK

FOOD	QTY	CALS	CARBS	PRO (g)	FAT (g)
	Sub Total				
	Total				

NUTRIENT	TOTAL	UNITS	GOAL %	RDA%
Calories				
Fat				
Saturated Fat				
Polyunsaturated				
Monounsaturated				

FOOD	QTY	CALS	CARBS	PRO (g)	FAT (g)

BREAKFAST

	Sub Total				

LUNCH

	Sub Total				

DINNER

	Sub Total				

SNACK

	Sub Total				
	Total				

NUTRIENT	TOTAL	UNITS	GOAL %	RDA%
Calories				
Fat				
Saturated Fat				
Polyunsaturated				
Monounsaturated				

FOOD	QTY	CALS	CARBS	PRO (g)	FAT (g)

BREAKFAST

	Sub Total				

LUNCH

	Sub Total				

DINNER

	Sub Total				

SNACK

	Sub Total				
	Total				

NUTRIENT	TOTAL	UNITS	GOAL %	RDA%
Calories				
Fat				
Saturated Fat				
Polyunsaturated				
Monounsaturated				

FOOD	QTY	CALS	CARBS	PRO (g)	FAT (g)

BREAKFAST

	Sub Total				

LUNCH

	Sub Total				

DINNER

	Sub Total				

SNACK

	Sub Total				
	Total				

NUTRIENT	TOTAL	UNITS	GOAL %	RDA%
Calories				
Fat				
Saturated Fat				
Polyunsaturated				
Monounsaturated				

FOOD	QTY	CALS	CARBS	PRO (g)	FAT (g)

BREAKFAST

	Sub Total				

LUNCH

	Sub Total				

DINNER

	Sub Total				

SNACK

	Sub Total				
	Total				

NUTRIENT	TOTAL	UNITS	GOAL %	RDA%
Calories				
Fat				
Saturated Fat				
Polyunsaturated				
Monounsaturated				

FOOD	QTY	CALS	CARBS	PRO (g)	FAT (g)

BREAKFAST

		Sub Total			

LUNCH

		Sub Total			

DINNER

		Sub Total			

SNACK

		Sub Total			
		Total			

NUTRIENT	TOTAL	UNITS	GOAL %	RDA%
Calories				
Fat				
Saturated Fat				
Polyunsaturated				
Monounsaturated				

FOOD	QTY	CALS	CARBS	PRO (g)	FAT (g)

BREAKFAST

	Sub Total				

LUNCH

	Sub Total				

DINNER

	Sub Total				

SNACK

	Sub Total				
	Total				

NUTRIENT	TOTAL	UNITS	GOAL %	RDA%
Calories				
Fat				
Saturated Fat				
Polyunsaturated				
Monounsaturated				

FOOD	QTY	CALS	CARBS	PRO (g)	FAT (g)

BREAKFAST

	Sub Total				

LUNCH

	Sub Total				

DINNER

	Sub Total				

SNACK

	Sub Total				
	Total				

NUTRIENT	TOTAL	UNITS	GOAL %	RDA%
Calories				
Fat				
Saturated Fat				
Polyunsaturated				
Monounsaturated				

FOOD	QTY	CALS	CARBS	PRO (g)	FAT (g)

BREAKFAST

	Sub Total				

LUNCH

	Sub Total				

DINNER

	Sub Total				

SNACK

	Sub Total				
	Total				

NUTRIENT	TOTAL	UNITS	GOAL %	RDA%
Calories				
Fat				
Saturated Fat				
Polyunsaturated				
Monounsaturated				

FOOD	QTY	CALS	CARBS	PRO (g)	FAT (g)

BREAKFAST

	Sub Total				

LUNCH

	Sub Total				

DINNER

	Sub Total				

SNACK

	Sub Total				
	Total				

NUTRIENT	TOTAL	UNITS	GOAL %	RDA%
Calories				
Fat				
Saturated Fat				
Polyunsaturated				
Monounsaturated				

FOOD	QTY	CALS	CARBS	PRO (g)	FAT (g)

BREAKFAST

	Sub Total				

LUNCH

	Sub Total				

DINNER

	Sub Total				

SNACK

	Sub Total				
	Total				

NUTRIENT	TOTAL	UNITS	GOAL %	RDA%
Calories				
Fat				
Saturated Fat				
Polyunsaturated				
Monounsaturated				

FOOD	QTY	CALS	CARBS	PRO (g)	FAT (g)

BREAKFAST

	Sub Total				

LUNCH

	Sub Total				

DINNER

	Sub Total				

SNACK

	Sub Total				
	Total				

NUTRIENT	TOTAL	UNITS	GOAL %	RDA%
Calories				
Fat				
Saturated Fat				
Polyunsaturated				
Monounsaturated				

FOOD	QTY	CALS	CARBS	PRO (g)	FAT (g)

BREAKFAST

	Sub Total				

LUNCH

	Sub Total				

DINNER

	Sub Total				

SNACK

	Sub Total				
	Total				

NUTRIENT	TOTAL	UNITS	GOAL %	RDA%
Calories				
Fat				
Saturated Fat				
Polyunsaturated				
Monounsaturated				

FOOD	QTY	CALS	CARBS	PRO (g)	FAT (g)

BREAKFAST

	Sub Total				

LUNCH

	Sub Total				

DINNER

	Sub Total				

SNACK

	Sub Total				
	Total				

NUTRIENT	TOTAL	UNITS	GOAL %	RDA%
Calories				
Fat				
Saturated Fat				
Polyunsaturated				
Monounsaturated				

FOOD	QTY	CALS	CARBS	PRO (g)	FAT (g)

BREAKFAST

	Sub Total				

LUNCH

	Sub Total				

DINNER

	Sub Total				

SNACK

	Sub Total				
	Total				

NUTRIENT	TOTAL	UNITS	GOAL %	RDA%
Calories				
Fat				
Saturated Fat				
Polyunsaturated				
Monounsaturated				

FOOD	QTY	CALS	CARBS	PRO (g)	FAT (g)

BREAKFAST

	Sub Total				

LUNCH

	Sub Total				

DINNER

	Sub Total				

SNACK

	Sub Total				
	Total				

NUTRIENT	TOTAL	UNITS	GOAL %	RDA%
Calories				
Fat				
Saturated Fat				
Polyunsaturated				
Monounsaturated				

FOOD	QTY	CALS	CARBS	PRO (g)	FAT (g)

BREAKFAST

	Sub Total				

LUNCH

	Sub Total				

DINNER

	Sub Total				

SNACK

	Sub Total				
	Total				

NUTRIENT	TOTAL	UNITS	GOAL %	RDA%
Calories				
Fat				
Saturated Fat				
Polyunsaturated				
Monounsaturated				

FOOD	QTY	CALS	CARBS	PRO (g)	FAT (g)

BREAKFAST

		Sub Total			

LUNCH

		Sub Total			

DINNER

		Sub Total			

SNACK

		Sub Total			
		Total			

NUTRIENT	TOTAL	UNITS	GOAL %	RDA%
Calories				
Fat				
Saturated Fat				
Polyunsaturated				
Monounsaturated				

FOOD	QTY	CALS	CARBS	PRO (g)	FAT (g)

BREAKFAST

	Sub Total				

LUNCH

	Sub Total				

DINNER

	Sub Total				

SNACK

	Sub Total				
	Total				

NUTRIENT	TOTAL	UNITS	GOAL %	RDA%
Calories				
Fat				
Saturated Fat				
Polyunsaturated				
Monounsaturated				

FOOD	QTY	CALS	CARBS	PRO (g)	FAT (g)

BREAKFAST

	Sub Total				

LUNCH

	Sub Total				

DINNER

	Sub Total				

SNACK

	Sub Total				
	Total				

NUTRIENT	TOTAL	UNITS	GOAL %	RDA%
Calories				
Fat				
Saturated Fat				
Polyunsaturated				
Monounsaturated				

FOOD	QTY	CALS	CARBS	PRO (g)	FAT (g)

BREAKFAST

FOOD	QTY	CALS	CARBS	PRO (g)	FAT (g)
	Sub Total				

LUNCH

FOOD	QTY	CALS	CARBS	PRO (g)	FAT (g)
	Sub Total				

DINNER

FOOD	QTY	CALS	CARBS	PRO (g)	FAT (g)
	Sub Total				

SNACK

FOOD	QTY	CALS	CARBS	PRO (g)	FAT (g)
	Sub Total				
	Total				

NUTRIENT	TOTAL	UNITS	GOAL %	RDA%
Calories				
Fat				
Saturated Fat				
Polyunsaturated				
Monounsaturated				

FOOD	QTY	CALS	CARBS	PRO (g)	FAT (g)

BREAKFAST

	Sub Total				

LUNCH

	Sub Total				

DINNER

	Sub Total				

SNACK

	Sub Total				
	Total				

NUTRIENT	TOTAL	UNITS	GOAL %	RDA%
Calories				
Fat				
Saturated Fat				
Polyunsaturated				
Monounsaturated				

FOOD	QTY	CALS	CARBS	PRO (g)	FAT (g)

BREAKFAST

	Sub Total				

LUNCH

	Sub Total				

DINNER

	Sub Total				

SNACK

	Sub Total				
	Total				

NUTRIENT	TOTAL	UNITS	GOAL %	RDA%
Calories				
Fat				
Saturated Fat				
Polyunsaturated				
Monounsaturated				

FOOD	QTY	CALS	CARBS	PRO (g)	FAT (g)

BREAKFAST

	Sub Total				

LUNCH

	Sub Total				

DINNER

	Sub Total				

SNACK

	Sub Total				
	Total				

NUTRIENT	TOTAL	UNITS	GOAL %	RDA%
Calories				
Fat				
Saturated Fat				
Polyunsaturated				
Monounsaturated				

FOOD	QTY	CALS	CARBS	PRO (g)	FAT (g)

BREAKFAST

	Sub Total				

LUNCH

	Sub Total				

DINNER

	Sub Total				

SNACK

	Sub Total				
	Total				

NUTRIENT	TOTAL	UNITS	GOAL %	RDA%
Calories				
Fat				
Saturated Fat				
Polyunsaturated				
Monounsaturated				

FOOD	QTY	CALS	CARBS	PRO (g)	FAT (g)

BREAKFAST

	Sub Total				

LUNCH

	Sub Total				

DINNER

	Sub Total				

SNACK

	Sub Total				
	Total				

NUTRIENT	TOTAL	UNITS	GOAL %	RDA%
Calories				
Fat				
Saturated Fat				
Polyunsaturated				
Monounsaturated				

FOOD	QTY	CALS	CARBS	PRO (g)	FAT (g)

BREAKFAST

		Sub Total			

LUNCH

		Sub Total			

DINNER

		Sub Total			

SNACK

		Sub Total			
		Total			

NUTRIENT	TOTAL	UNITS	GOAL %	RDA%
Calories				
Fat				
Saturated Fat				
Polyunsaturated				
Monounsaturated				

FOOD	QTY	CALS	CARBS	PRO (g)	FAT (g)

BREAKFAST

	Sub Total				

LUNCH

	Sub Total				

DINNER

	Sub Total				

SNACK

	Sub Total				
	Total				

NUTRIENT	TOTAL	UNITS	GOAL %	RDA%
Calories				
Fat				
Saturated Fat				
Polyunsaturated				
Monounsaturated				

FOOD	QTY	CALS	CARBS	PRO (g)	FAT (g)

BREAKFAST

	Sub Total				

LUNCH

	Sub Total				

DINNER

	Sub Total				

SNACK

	Sub Total				
	Total				

NUTRIENT	TOTAL	UNITS	GOAL %	RDA%
Calories				
Fat				
Saturated Fat				
Polyunsaturated				
Monounsaturated				

FOOD	QTY	CALS	CARBS	PRO (g)	FAT (g)

BREAKFAST

	Sub Total				

LUNCH

	Sub Total				

DINNER

	Sub Total				

SNACK

	Sub Total				
	Total				

NUTRIENT	TOTAL	UNITS	GOAL %	RDA%
Calories				
Fat				
Saturated Fat				
Polyunsaturated				
Monounsaturated				

FOOD	QTY	CALS	CARBS	PRO (g)	FAT (g)

BREAKFAST

	Sub Total				

LUNCH

	Sub Total				

DINNER

	Sub Total				

SNACK

	Sub Total				
	Total				

NUTRIENT	TOTAL	UNITS	GOAL %	RDA%
Calories				
Fat				
Saturated Fat				
Polyunsaturated				
Monounsaturated				

FOOD	QTY	CALS	CARBS	PRO (g)	FAT (g)

BREAKFAST

		Sub Total			

LUNCH

		Sub Total			

DINNER

		Sub Total			

SNACK

		Sub Total			
		Total			

NUTRIENT	TOTAL	UNITS	GOAL %	RDA%
Calories				
Fat				
Saturated Fat				
Polyunsaturated				
Monounsaturated				

FOOD	QTY	CALS	CARBS	PRO (g)	FAT (g)

BREAKFAST

FOOD	QTY	CALS	CARBS	PRO (g)	FAT (g)
	Sub Total				

LUNCH

FOOD	QTY	CALS	CARBS	PRO (g)	FAT (g)
	Sub Total				

DINNER

FOOD	QTY	CALS	CARBS	PRO (g)	FAT (g)
	Sub Total				

SNACK

FOOD	QTY	CALS	CARBS	PRO (g)	FAT (g)
	Sub Total				
	Total				

NUTRIENT	TOTAL	UNITS	GOAL %	RDA%
Calories				
Fat				
Saturated Fat				
Polyunsaturated				
Monounsaturated				

FOOD	QTY	CALS	CARBS	PRO (g)	FAT (g)

BREAKFAST

FOOD	QTY	CALS	CARBS	PRO (g)	FAT (g)
	Sub Total				

LUNCH

FOOD	QTY	CALS	CARBS	PRO (g)	FAT (g)
	Sub Total				

DINNER

FOOD	QTY	CALS	CARBS	PRO (g)	FAT (g)
	Sub Total				

SNACK

FOOD	QTY	CALS	CARBS	PRO (g)	FAT (g)
	Sub Total				
	Total				

NUTRIENT	TOTAL	UNITS	GOAL %	RDA%
Calories				
Fat				
Saturated Fat				
Polyunsaturated				
Monounsaturated				

FOOD	QTY	CALS	CARBS	PRO (g)	FAT (g)

BREAKFAST

FOOD	QTY	CALS	CARBS	PRO (g)	FAT (g)
	Sub Total				

LUNCH

FOOD	QTY	CALS	CARBS	PRO (g)	FAT (g)
	Sub Total				

DINNER

FOOD	QTY	CALS	CARBS	PRO (g)	FAT (g)
	Sub Total				

SNACK

FOOD	QTY	CALS	CARBS	PRO (g)	FAT (g)
	Sub Total				
	Total				

NUTRIENT	TOTAL	UNITS	GOAL %	RDA%
Calories				
Fat				
Saturated Fat				
Polyunsaturated				
Monounsaturated				

FOOD	QTY	CALS	CARBS	PRO (g)	FAT (g)

BREAKFAST

	Sub Total				

LUNCH

	Sub Total				

DINNER

	Sub Total				

SNACK

	Sub Total				
	Total				

NUTRIENT	TOTAL	UNITS	GOAL %	RDA%
Calories				
Fat				
Saturated Fat				
Polyunsaturated				
Monounsaturated				

FOOD	QTY	CALS	CARBS	PRO (g)	FAT (g)

BREAKFAST

	Sub Total				

LUNCH

	Sub Total				

DINNER

	Sub Total				

SNACK

	Sub Total				
	Total				

NUTRIENT	TOTAL	UNITS	GOAL %	RDA%
Calories				
Fat				
Saturated Fat				
Polyunsaturated				
Monounsaturated				

FOOD	QTY	CALS	CARBS	PRO (g)	FAT (g)

BREAKFAST

	Sub Total				

LUNCH

	Sub Total				

DINNER

	Sub Total				

SNACK

	Sub Total				
	Total				

NUTRIENT	TOTAL	UNITS	GOAL %	RDA%
Calories				
Fat				
Saturated Fat				
Polyunsaturated				
Monounsaturated				

FOOD	QTY	CALS	CARBS	PRO (g)	FAT (g)

BREAKFAST

	Sub Total				

LUNCH

	Sub Total				

DINNER

	Sub Total				

SNACK

	Sub Total				
	Total				

NUTRIENT	TOTAL	UNITS	GOAL %	RDA%
Calories				
Fat				
Saturated Fat				
Polyunsaturated				
Monounsaturated				

FOOD	QTY	CALS	CARBS	PRO (g)	FAT (g)

BREAKFAST

	Sub Total				

LUNCH

	Sub Total				

DINNER

	Sub Total				

SNACK

	Sub Total				
	Total				

NUTRIENT	TOTAL	UNITS	GOAL %	RDA%
Calories				
Fat				
Saturated Fat				
Polyunsaturated				
Monounsaturated				

FOOD	QTY	CALS	CARBS	PRO (g)	FAT (g)
BREAKFAST					
Sub Total					
LUNCH					
Sub Total					
DINNER					
Sub Total					
SNACK					
Sub Total					
Total					

NUTRIENT	TOTAL	UNITS	GOAL %	RDA%
Calories				
Fat				
Saturated Fat				
Polyunsaturated				
Monounsaturated				

FOOD	QTY	CALS	CARBS	PRO (g)	FAT (g)

BREAKFAST

FOOD	QTY	CALS	CARBS	PRO (g)	FAT (g)
	Sub Total				

LUNCH

FOOD	QTY	CALS	CARBS	PRO (g)	FAT (g)
	Sub Total				

DINNER

FOOD	QTY	CALS	CARBS	PRO (g)	FAT (g)
	Sub Total				

SNACK

FOOD	QTY	CALS	CARBS	PRO (g)	FAT (g)
	Sub Total				
	Total				

NUTRIENT	TOTAL	UNITS	GOAL %	RDA%
Calories				
Fat				
Saturated Fat				
Polyunsaturated				
Monounsaturated				

FOOD	QTY	CALS	CARBS	PRO (g)	FAT (g)

BREAKFAST

	Sub Total				

LUNCH

	Sub Total				

DINNER

	Sub Total				

SNACK

	Sub Total				
	Total				

NUTRIENT	TOTAL	UNITS	GOAL %	RDA%
Calories				
Fat				
Saturated Fat				
Polyunsaturated				
Monounsaturated				

FOOD	QTY	CALS	CARBS	PRO (g)	FAT (g)

BREAKFAST

	Sub Total				

LUNCH

	Sub Total				

DINNER

	Sub Total				

SNACK

	Sub Total				
	Total				

NUTRIENT	TOTAL	UNITS	GOAL %	RDA%
Calories				
Fat				
Saturated Fat				
Polyunsaturated				
Monounsaturated				

FOOD	QTY	CALS	CARBS	PRO (g)	FAT (g)

BREAKFAST

Sub Total					

LUNCH

Sub Total					

DINNER

Sub Total					

SNACK

Sub Total					
Total					

NUTRIENT	TOTAL	UNITS	GOAL %	RDA%
Calories				
Fat				
Saturated Fat				
Polyunsaturated				
Monounsaturated				

FOOD	QTY	CALS	CARBS	PRO (g)	FAT (g)

BREAKFAST

	Sub Total				

LUNCH

	Sub Total				

DINNER

	Sub Total				

SNACK

	Sub Total				
	Total				

NUTRIENT	TOTAL	UNITS	GOAL %	RDA%
Calories				
Fat				
Saturated Fat				
Polyunsaturated				
Monounsaturated				

FOOD	QTY	CALS	CARBS	PRO (g)	FAT (g)

BREAKFAST

	Sub Total				

LUNCH

	Sub Total				

DINNER

	Sub Total				

SNACK

	Sub Total				
	Total				

NUTRIENT	TOTAL	UNITS	GOAL %	RDA%
Calories				
Fat				
Saturated Fat				
Polyunsaturated				
Monounsaturated				

FOOD	QTY	CALS	CARBS	PRO (g)	FAT (g)

BREAKFAST

	Sub Total				

LUNCH

	Sub Total				

DINNER

	Sub Total				

SNACK

	Sub Total				
	Total				

NUTRIENT	TOTAL	UNITS	GOAL %	RDA%
Calories				
Fat				
Saturated Fat				
Polyunsaturated				
Monounsaturated				

FOOD	QTY	CALS	CARBS	PRO (g)	FAT (g)

BREAKFAST

FOOD	QTY	CALS	CARBS	PRO (g)	FAT (g)
	Sub Total				

LUNCH

FOOD	QTY	CALS	CARBS	PRO (g)	FAT (g)
	Sub Total				

DINNER

FOOD	QTY	CALS	CARBS	PRO (g)	FAT (g)
	Sub Total				

SNACK

FOOD	QTY	CALS	CARBS	PRO (g)	FAT (g)
	Sub Total				
	Total				

NUTRIENT	TOTAL	UNITS	GOAL %	RDA%
Calories				
Fat				
Saturated Fat				
Polyunsaturated				
Monounsaturated				

FOOD	QTY	CALS	CARBS	PRO (g)	FAT (g)

BREAKFAST

	Sub Total				

LUNCH

	Sub Total				

DINNER

	Sub Total				

SNACK

	Sub Total				
	Total				

NUTRIENT	TOTAL	UNITS	GOAL %	RDA%
Calories				
Fat				
Saturated Fat				
Polyunsaturated				
Monounsaturated				

FOOD	QTY	CALS	CARBS	PRO (g)	FAT (g)

BREAKFAST

	Sub Total				

LUNCH

	Sub Total				

DINNER

	Sub Total				

SNACK

	Sub Total				
	Total				

NUTRIENT	TOTAL	UNITS	GOAL %	RDA%
Calories				
Fat				
Saturated Fat				
Polyunsaturated				
Monounsaturated				

FOOD	QTY	CALS	CARBS	PRO (g)	FAT (g)

BREAKFAST

	Sub Total				

LUNCH

	Sub Total				

DINNER

	Sub Total				

SNACK

	Sub Total				
	Total				

NUTRIENT	TOTAL	UNITS	GOAL %	RDA%
Calories				
Fat				
Saturated Fat				
Polyunsaturated				
Monounsaturated				

FOOD	QTY	CALS	CARBS	PRO (g)	FAT (g)

BREAKFAST

	Sub Total				

LUNCH

	Sub Total				

DINNER

	Sub Total				

SNACK

	Sub Total				
	Total				

NUTRIENT	TOTAL	UNITS	GOAL %	RDA%
Calories				
Fat				
Saturated Fat				
Polyunsaturated				
Monounsaturated				

FOOD	QTY	CALS	CARBS	PRO (g)	FAT (g)

BREAKFAST

	Sub Total				

LUNCH

	Sub Total				

DINNER

	Sub Total				

SNACK

	Sub Total				
	Total				

NUTRIENT	TOTAL	UNITS	GOAL %	RDA%
Calories				
Fat				
Saturated Fat				
Polyunsaturated				
Monounsaturated				

FOOD	QTY	CALS	CARBS	PRO (g)	FAT (g)

BREAKFAST

FOOD	QTY	CALS	CARBS	PRO (g)	FAT (g)
	Sub Total				

LUNCH

FOOD	QTY	CALS	CARBS	PRO (g)	FAT (g)
	Sub Total				

DINNER

FOOD	QTY	CALS	CARBS	PRO (g)	FAT (g)
	Sub Total				

SNACK

FOOD	QTY	CALS	CARBS	PRO (g)	FAT (g)
	Sub Total				
	Total				

NUTRIENT	TOTAL	UNITS	GOAL %	RDA%
Calories				
Fat				
Saturated Fat				
Polyunsaturated				
Monounsaturated				

FOOD	QTY	CALS	CARBS	PRO (g)	FAT (g)

BREAKFAST

FOOD	QTY	CALS	CARBS	PRO (g)	FAT (g)
	Sub Total				

LUNCH

FOOD	QTY	CALS	CARBS	PRO (g)	FAT (g)
	Sub Total				

DINNER

FOOD	QTY	CALS	CARBS	PRO (g)	FAT (g)
	Sub Total				

SNACK

FOOD	QTY	CALS	CARBS	PRO (g)	FAT (g)
	Sub Total				
	Total				

NUTRIENT	TOTAL	UNITS	GOAL %	RDA%
Calories				
Fat				
Saturated Fat				
Polyunsaturated				
Monounsaturated				

FOOD	QTY	CALS	CARBS	PRO (g)	FAT (g)

BREAKFAST

	Sub Total				

LUNCH

	Sub Total				

DINNER

	Sub Total				

SNACK

	Sub Total				
	Total				

NUTRIENT	TOTAL	UNITS	GOAL %	RDA%
Calories				
Fat				
Saturated Fat				
Polyunsaturated				
Monounsaturated				

FOOD	QTY	CALS	CARBS	PRO (g)	FAT (g)

BREAKFAST

FOOD	QTY	CALS	CARBS	PRO (g)	FAT (g)
	Sub Total				

LUNCH

FOOD	QTY	CALS	CARBS	PRO (g)	FAT (g)
	Sub Total				

DINNER

FOOD	QTY	CALS	CARBS	PRO (g)	FAT (g)
	Sub Total				

SNACK

FOOD	QTY	CALS	CARBS	PRO (g)	FAT (g)
	Sub Total				
	Total				

NUTRIENT	TOTAL	UNITS	GOAL %	RDA%
Calories				
Fat				
Saturated Fat				
Polyunsaturated				
Monounsaturated				

FOOD	QTY	CALS	CARBS	PRO (g)	FAT (g)

BREAKFAST

	Sub Total				

LUNCH

	Sub Total				

DINNER

	Sub Total				

SNACK

	Sub Total				
	Total				

NUTRIENT	TOTAL	UNITS	GOAL %	RDA%
Calories				
Fat				
Saturated Fat				
Polyunsaturated				
Monounsaturated				

FOOD	QTY	CALS	CARBS	PRO (g)	FAT (g)

BREAKFAST

FOOD	QTY	CALS	CARBS	PRO (g)	FAT (g)
	Sub Total				

LUNCH

FOOD	QTY	CALS	CARBS	PRO (g)	FAT (g)
	Sub Total				

DINNER

FOOD	QTY	CALS	CARBS	PRO (g)	FAT (g)
	Sub Total				

SNACK

FOOD	QTY	CALS	CARBS	PRO (g)	FAT (g)
	Sub Total				
	Total				

NUTRIENT	TOTAL	UNITS	GOAL %	RDA%
Calories				
Fat				
Saturated Fat				
Polyunsaturated				
Monounsaturated				

FOOD	QTY	CALS	CARBS	PRO (g)	FAT (g)

BREAKFAST

	Sub Total				

LUNCH

	Sub Total				

DINNER

	Sub Total				

SNACK

	Sub Total				
	Total				

NUTRIENT	TOTAL	UNITS	GOAL %	RDA%
Calories				
Fat				
Saturated Fat				
Polyunsaturated				
Monounsaturated				

FOOD	QTY	CALS	CARBS	PRO (g)	FAT (g)

BREAKFAST

FOOD	QTY	CALS	CARBS	PRO (g)	FAT (g)
Sub Total					

LUNCH

FOOD	QTY	CALS	CARBS	PRO (g)	FAT (g)
Sub Total					

DINNER

FOOD	QTY	CALS	CARBS	PRO (g)	FAT (g)
Sub Total					

SNACK

FOOD	QTY	CALS	CARBS	PRO (g)	FAT (g)
Sub Total					
Total					

NUTRIENT	TOTAL	UNITS	GOAL %	RDA%
Calories				
Fat				
Saturated Fat				
Polyunsaturated				
Monounsaturated				

FOOD	QTY	CALS	CARBS	PRO (g)	FAT (g)

BREAKFAST

	Sub Total				

LUNCH

	Sub Total				

DINNER

	Sub Total				

SNACK

	Sub Total				
	Total				

NUTRIENT	TOTAL	UNITS	GOAL %	RDA%
Calories				
Fat				
Saturated Fat				
Polyunsaturated				
Monounsaturated				

FOOD	QTY	CALS	CARBS	PRO (g)	FAT (g)

BREAKFAST

		Sub Total			

LUNCH

		Sub Total			

DINNER

		Sub Total			

SNACK

		Sub Total			
		Total			

NUTRIENT	TOTAL	UNITS	GOAL %	RDA%
Calories				
Fat				
Saturated Fat				
Polyunsaturated				
Monounsaturated				

FOOD	QTY	CALS	CARBS	PRO (g)	FAT (g)

BREAKFAST

	Sub Total				

LUNCH

	Sub Total				

DINNER

	Sub Total				

SNACK

	Sub Total				
	Total				

NUTRIENT	TOTAL	UNITS	GOAL %	RDA%
Calories				
Fat				
Saturated Fat				
Polyunsaturated				
Monounsaturated				

FOOD	QTY	CALS	CARBS	PRO (g)	FAT (g)

BREAKFAST

		Sub Total			

LUNCH

		Sub Total			

DINNER

		Sub Total			

SNACK

		Sub Total			
		Total			

NUTRIENT	TOTAL	UNITS	GOAL %	RDA%
Calories				
Fat				
Saturated Fat				
Polyunsaturated				
Monounsaturated